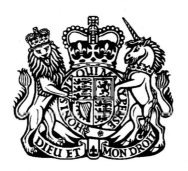

Equity and excellence: Liberating the NHS

Presented to Parliament
by the Secretary of State for Health
by Command of Her Majesty

July 2010

Cm 7881

ISBN: 9780101788120

Printed in the UK by The Stationery Office Limited
on behalf of the Controller of Her Majesty's Stationery Office

ID P002377484   07/10

Foreword

The NHS is a great national institution. The principles it was founded on are as important now as they were then: free at the point of use and available to everyone based on need, not ability to pay. But we believe that it can be so much better – for both patients and professionals.

That's why we've set out a bold vision for the future of the NHS - rooted in the coalition's core beliefs of freedom, fairness and responsibility.

We will make the NHS more accountable to patients. We will free staff from excessive bureaucracy and top-down control. We will increase real terms spending on the health service in every year of this Parliament.

Our ambition is to once again make the NHS the envy of the world. *Liberating the NHS* - a blend of Conservative and Liberal Democrat ideas - sets out our plans to do this.

First, patients will be at the heart of everything we do. So they will have more choice and control, helped by easy access to the information they need about the best GPs and hospitals. Patients will be in charge of making decisions about their care.

Second, there will be a relentless focus on clinical outcomes. Success will be measured, not through bureaucratic process targets, but against results that really matter to patients – such as improving cancer and stroke survival rates.

Third, we will empower health professionals. Doctors and nurses must to be able to use their professional judgement about what is right for patients. We will support this by giving front-line staff more control. Healthcare will be run from the bottom up, with ownership and decision-making in the hands of professionals and patients.

Of course, our massive deficit and growing debt means there are some difficult decisions to make. The NHS is not immune from those challenges. But far from that being reason to abandon reform, it demands that we accelerate it. Only by putting patients first and trusting professionals will we drive up standards, deliver better value for money and create a healthier nation.

Prime Minister   **Deputy Prime Minister**

Secretary of State for Health

Contents

Our strategy for the NHS: an executive summary

1.   The Government upholds the values and principles of the NHS: of a comprehensive service, available to all, free at the point of use and based on clinical need, not the ability to pay.

2.   We will increase health spending in real terms in each year of this Parliament.

3.   Our goal is an NHS which achieves results that are amongst the best in the world.

Putting patients and public first

4.   We will put patients at the heart of the NHS, through an information revolution and greater choice and control:

   a.   Shared decision-making will become the norm: *no decision about me without me*.

   b.   Patients will have access to the information they want, to make choices about their care. They will have increased control over their own care records.

   c.   Patients will have choice of any provider, choice of consultant-led team, choice of GP practice and choice of treatment. We will extend choice in maternity through new maternity networks.

   d.   The Government will enable patients to rate hospitals and clinical departments according to the quality of care they receive, and we will require hospitals to be open about mistakes and always tell patients if something has gone wrong.

   e.   The system will focus on personalised care that reflects individuals' health and care needs, supports carers and encourages strong joint arrangements and local partnerships.

   f.   We will strengthen the collective voice of patients and the public through arrangements led by local authorities, and at national level, through a powerful new consumer champion, HealthWatch England, located in the Care Quality Commission.

   g.   We will seek to ensure that everyone, whatever their need or background, benefits from these arrangements.

Improving healthcare outcomes

5.   To achieve our ambition for world-class healthcare outcomes, the service must be focused on outcomes and the quality standards that deliver them. The Government's objectives are to reduce mortality and morbidity, increase safety, and improve patient experience and outcomes for all:

h.   The NHS will be held to account against clinically credible and evidence-based outcome measures, not process targets. We will remove targets with no clinical justification.

i.   A culture of open information, active responsibility and challenge will ensure that patient safety is put above all else, and that failings such as those in Mid-Staffordshire cannot go undetected.

j.   Quality standards, developed by NICE, will inform the commissioning of all NHS care and payment systems. Inspection will be against essential quality standards.

k.   We will pay drug companies according to the value of new medicines, to promote innovation, ensure better access for patients to effective drugs and improve value for money. As an interim measure, we are creating a new Cancer Drug Fund, which will operate from April 2011; this fund will support patients to get the drugs their doctors recommend.

l.   Money will follow the patient through transparent, comprehensive and stable payment systems across the NHS to promote high quality care, drive efficiency, and support patient choice.

m.   Providers will be paid according to their performance. Payment should reflect outcomes, not just activity, and provide an incentive for better quality.

Autonomy, accountability and democratic legitimacy

6. The Government's reforms will empower professionals and providers, giving them more autonomy and, in return, making them more accountable for the results they achieve, accountable to patients through choice and accountable to the public at local level:

n.   The forthcoming Health Bill will give the NHS greater freedoms and help prevent political micromanagement.

o.   The Government will devolve power and responsibility for commissioning services to the healthcare professionals closest to patients: GPs and their practice teams working in consortia.

p.   To strengthen democratic legitimacy at local level, local authorities will promote the joining up of local NHS services, social care and health improvement.

q. We will establish an independent and accountable NHS Commissioning Board. The Board will lead on the achievement of health outcomes, allocate and account for NHS resources, lead on quality improvement and promoting patient involvement and choice. The Board will have an explicit duty to promote equality and tackle inequalities in access to healthcare. We will limit the powers of Ministers over day-to-day NHS decisions.

r. We aim to create the largest social enterprise sector in the world by increasing the freedoms of foundation trusts and giving NHS staff the opportunity to have a greater say in the future of their organisations, including as employee-led social enterprises. All NHS trusts will become or be part of a foundation trust.

s. Monitor will become an economic regulator, to promote effective and efficient providers of health and care, to promote competition, regulate prices and safeguard the continuity of services.

t. We will strengthen the role of the Care Quality Commission as an effective quality inspectorate across both health and social care.

u. We will ring-fence the public health budget, allocated to reflect relative population health outcomes, with a new health premium to promote action to reduce health inequalities.

Cutting bureaucracy and improving efficiency

7. The NHS will need to achieve unprecedented efficiency gains, with savings reinvested in front-line services, to meet the current financial challenge and the future costs of demographic and technological change:

v. The NHS will release up to £20 billion of efficiency savings by 2014, which will be reinvested to support improvements in quality and outcomes.

w. The Government will reduce NHS management costs by more than 45% over the next four years, freeing up further resources for front-line care.

x. We will radically delayer and simplify the number of NHS bodies, and radically reduce the Department of Health's own NHS functions. We will abolish quangos that do not need to exist and streamline the functions of those that do.

Conclusion: making it happen

8. We will maintain constancy of purpose. This White Paper[1] is the long-term plan for the NHS in this Parliamentary term and beyond. We will give the NHS a coherent, stable, enduring framework for quality and service improvement. The debate on health should

no longer be about structures and processes, but about priorities and progress in health improvement for all.

9. This is a challenging and far-reaching set of reforms, which will drive cultural changes in the NHS. We are setting out plans for managing change, including the transitional roles of strategic health authorities and primary care trusts. Implementation will happen bottom-up.

Many of the commitments made in this White Paper require primary legislation and are subject to Parliamentary approval.

1.   Liberating the NHS

Our values

1.1   It is our privilege to be custodians of the NHS, its values and principles. We believe that the NHS is an integral part of a Big Society, reflecting the social solidarity of shared access to collective healthcare, and a shared responsibility to use resources effectively to deliver better health.

1.2   We are committed to an NHS that is available to all, free at the point of use, and based on need, not the ability to pay. We will increase health spending in real terms in each year of this Parliament.

1.3   The NHS is about fairness for everyone in our society. It is about this country doing the right thing for those who need help. We are committed to promoting equality[2] and will implement the ban on age discrimination in NHS services and social care to take effect from 2012. The NHS Commissioning Board will have an explicit duty to address inequalities in outcomes from healthcare services.

1.4   We will uphold the NHS Constitution, the development of which enjoyed cross-party support. By 2012, the Government will publish the first statement of how well organisations are living by its letter and spirit.[3] The NHS Constitution codifies NHS principles and values, and the rights and responsibilities of patients and staff. It is about mutuality; and our proposals in chapter 2 for shared decision-making by patients, their carers, and clinicians will give better effect to this principle. It is also about NHS-funded organisations being good employers; and our plans in chapter 4 will give organisations and professionals greater freedoms, leading to better staff engagement and better patient care.

1.5   Current statutory arrangements allow the Secretary of State a large amount of discretion to micromanage parts of the NHS.[4] We will be clear about what the NHS should achieve; we will not prescribe how it should be achieved. We will legislate to establish more autonomous NHS institutions, with greater freedoms, clear duties, and transparency in their responsibilities to patients and their accountabilities. We will use our powers in order to devolve them.

The NHS today

1.6   At its best, the NHS is world-class. The people who work in the NHS are among the most talented in the world, and some of the most dedicated public servants in the country. Other countries seek to learn from our comprehensive system of general practice, and its role as the medical home for patients, providing continuity of care and coordination. The NHS has an increasingly strong focus on evidence-based medicine, supported by internationally respected clinical researchers with funding from the National Institute for Health Research, and the National Institute for Health and Clinical Excellence (NICE). Other countries admire NHS delivery of immunisation programmes. Our patient participation levels in cancer research are the highest in the world.[5]

1.7 We will build on the ongoing good work in the NHS. We recognise the importance of Lord Darzi's work, in putting a stronger emphasis on quality.

1.8 Compared to other countries, however, the NHS has achieved relatively poor outcomes in some areas. For example, rates of mortality amenable to healthcare,[6] rates of mortality from some respiratory diseases and some cancers,[7] and some measures of stroke[8] have been amongst the worst in the developed world.[9] In part this is due to differences in underlying risk factors, which is why we need to re-focus on public health. But international evidence also shows we have much further to go on managing care more effectively. For example, the NHS has high rates of acute complications of diabetes and avoidable asthma admissions;[10] the incidence of MRSA infection has been worse than the European average;[11] and venous thromboembolism causes 25,000 avoidable deaths each year.[12]

1.9 The NHS also scores relatively poorly on being responsive to the patients it serves. It lacks a genuinely patient-centred approach in which services are designed around individual needs, lifestyles and aspirations. Too often, patients are expected to fit around services, rather than services around patients. The NHS is admired for the equity in access to healthcare it achieves; but not for the consistency of excellence to which we aspire. Our intention is to secure excellence as well as equity.

Our vision for the NHS

1.10 We can foresee a better NHS that:

- **Is genuinely centred on patients and carers;**

- **Achieves quality and outcomes that are among the best in the world;**

- **Refuses to tolerate unsafe and substandard care;**

- **Eliminates discrimination and reduces inequalities in care;**

- **Puts clinicians in the driving seat and sets hospitals and providers free to innovate, with stronger incentives to adopt best practice;**

- **Is more transparent, with clearer accountabilities for quality and results;**

- **Gives citizens a greater say in how the NHS is run;**

- **Is less insular and fragmented, and works much better across boundaries, including with local authorities and between hospitals and practices;**

- **Is more efficient and dynamic, with a radically smaller national, regional and local bureaucracy; and**

- **Is put on a more stable and sustainable footing, free from frequent and arbitrary political meddling.**

1.11   This is our vision. It is based on our commitment to NHS values and principles, and is about building on what is best in the NHS today, and striving for continual improvement, while being open and honest about shortcomings. Our strategy to implement this vision draws inspiration from the coalition principles of freedom, fairness and responsibility[13].

1.12   The headquarters of the NHS will not be in the Department of Health or the new NHS Commissioning Board but instead, power will be given to the front-line clinicians and patients. The headquarters will be in the consulting room and clinic. The Government will liberate the NHS from excessive bureaucratic and political control, and make it easier for professionals to do the right things for and with patients, to innovate and improve outcomes. We will create an environment where staff and organisations enjoy greater freedom and clearer incentives to flourish, but also know the consequences of failing the patients they serve and the taxpayers who fund them.

1.13   The current architecture of the health system has developed piecemeal, involves duplication, and is unwieldy. Liberating the NHS, and putting power in the hands of patients and clinicians, means we will be able to effect a radical simplification, and remove layers of management. We will build on key aspects of the existing arrangements: for example, a number of GP consortia are likely to emerge from practice-based commissioning clusters and Monitor will become the economic regulator.

Improving public health and reforming social care

1.14   Liberating the NHS will fundamentally change the role of the Department. Its NHS role will be much reduced and more strategic. It will focus on improving public health, tackling health inequalities and reforming adult social care.

1.15   We will set out our programme for public health in a White Paper later this year. The forthcoming Health Bill will support the creation of a new Public Health Service, to integrate and streamline existing health improvement and protection bodies and functions, including an increased emphasis on research, analysis and evaluation. It will be responsible for vaccination and screening programmes and, in order to manage public health emergencies, it will have powers in relation to the NHS matched by corresponding duties for NHS resilience.

1.16 PCT responsibilities for local health improvement will transfer to local authorities, who will employ the Director of Public Health jointly appointed with the Public Health Service. The Department will create a ring-fenced public health budget and, within this, local Directors of Public Health will be responsible for health improvement funds allocated according to relative population health need. The allocation formula for those funds will include a new "health premium" designed to promote action to improve population-wide health and reduce health inequalities.

1.17 The Department will continue to have a vital role in setting adult social care policy. We want a sustainable adult social care system that gives people support and freedom to lead the life they choose, with dignity. We recognise the critical interdependence between the NHS and the adult social care system in securing better outcomes for people, including carers. We will seek to break down barriers between health and social care funding to encourage preventative action. Later this year we will set out our vision for adult social care, to enable people to have greater control over their care and support so they can enjoy maximum independence and responsibility for their own lives. The Department will continue to work closely with the Department for Education on services for children, to ensure that the changes in this White Paper and the subsequent public health White Paper support local health, education and social care services to work together for children and families.

1.18 The Department will establish a commission on the funding of long-term care and support, to report within a year. We understand the urgency of reforming the system of funding social care. The Commission will consider a range of ideas, including both a voluntary insurance scheme and a partnership scheme. As a key component of a lasting settlement for the social care system, we will reform and consolidate the law underpinning adult social care, working with the Law Commission.

1.19 The Government will bring together the conclusions of the Law Commission and the Commission on funding of long-term care, along with our vision, into a White Paper in 2011, with a view to introducing legislation in the second session of this Parliament to establish a sustainable legal and financial framework for adult social care.

The financial position

1.20 We know that the reforms that we are proposing in this White Paper will take place against the backdrop of a very challenging financial position. In the Coalition Agreement, the Government said that the single greatest priority for the next Parliament will be to reduce the deficit. It is now even more pressing that we implement the reforms set out here in order to increase productivity and efficiency in the NHS.

1.21 We will increase NHS spending in real terms in each year of this Parliament. Despite this, local NHS organisations will need to achieve unprecedented efficiency gains, if we are to meet the costs of demographic and technological changes, and even more so if we are to achieve quality and improve outcomes. Large cuts in administrative costs will provide an important but still modest contribution. In the next five years, the NHS will only be able to increase quality through implementing best practice and increasing productivity. This will be difficult work. Inevitably, as a result of the record debt, the NHS will employ fewer staff at the end of this Parliament; although rebalanced towards clinical staffing and front-line support rather than excessive administration. This is a hard truth which any government would have to recognise.

1.22 All of this means we have a responsibility to ensure that funding is used as efficiently as possible. The proposals laid out in this White Paper are a part of this. They are intended to put the NHS onto a sustainable footing, so that everyone in the system – from the Department to groups of GP practices – is accountable for the best use of funding. We are very clear that there will be no bail-outs for organisations which overspend public budgets.

Implementing our NHS vision

1.23 Our strategy is about making changes for the long-term; not just for this Parliament, but beyond. Experience in other sectors and abroad shows that embedding change takes time, and requires ongoing adaptation. The Department is committed to evidence-based policy-making and a culture of evaluation and learning.

1.24 Many will welcome our vision and clarity of intention, our insistence on transparency, and our sense of real urgency. Others may find it too challenging. Throughout, we will maintain constancy of purpose. This White Paper is our strategy for the NHS during this Parliamentary term, so that it is liberated to deliver the best quality care over the longer-term. In the next five years, the coalition Government will not produce another long-term plan for the NHS.

1.25 The NHS will face very significant challenges along the way. The new financial context will require difficult local decisions in the NHS, irrespective of this White Paper.[14] We will be open and honest about what this means.

1.26 These reforms will make the NHS more responsive and transparent, better able to withstand the funding pressures of the future. Once they are in place, it will not just be the responsibility of government, but of every commissioner, every healthcare provider and every GP practice to ensure that taxpayers' money is used to achieve the best possible outcomes for patients.

1.27   The following chapters set out how we will bring about this long-term transformation through:

- putting patients and the public first;

- focusing on improvement in quality and healthcare outcomes;

- autonomy, accountability and democratic legitimacy; and

- cutting bureaucracy and improving efficiency.

1.28   These plans are interconnected and mutually reinforcing. The final chapter sets out plans for making it happen. The Department will take forward work to manage the transition and flesh out further policy details in partnership with external organisations, seeking their help and expertise.

2. Putting patients and the public first

Shared decision making: nothing about me without me

2.1 The Government's ambition is to achieve healthcare outcomes that are among the best in the world. This can only be realised by involving patients fully in their own care, with decisions made in partnership with clinicians, rather than by clinicians alone.

2.2 Healthcare outcomes are personal to each of us. The outcomes we experience reflect the quality of our interaction with the professionals that serve us.[15] But compared to other sectors, healthcare systems are in their infancy in putting the experience of the user first, and have barely started to realise the potential of patients as joint providers of their own care and recovery. Progress has been limited in making the NHS truly patient led.[16] We intend to put that right.

2.3 We want the principle of "shared decision-making" to become the norm: *no decision about me without me*. International evidence shows that involving patients in their care and treatment improves their health outcomes,[17] boosts their satisfaction with services received, and increases not just their knowledge and understanding of their health status but also their adherence to a chosen treatment.[18] It can also bring significant reductions in cost, as highlighted in the Wanless Report,[19] and in evidence from various programmes to improve the management of long-term conditions.[20] This is equally true of the partnership between patients and clinicians in research, where those institutions with strong participation in clinical trials tend to have better outcomes.

2.4 The new NHS Commissioning Board will champion patient and carer involvement, and the Secretary of State will hold it to account for progress. In the meantime, the Department will work with patients, carers and professional groups, to bring forward proposals about transforming care through shared decision-making.

An NHS information revolution

2.5 Information, combined with the right support, is the key to better care, better outcomes and reduced costs. Patients need and should have far more information and data on all aspects of healthcare, to enable them to share in decisions made about their care and find out much more easily about services that are available.

2.6 The Government intends to bring about an NHS information revolution, to correct the imbalance in who knows what. Our aim is to give people access to comprehensive, trustworthy and easy to understand information from a range of sources on conditions, treatments, lifestyle choices and how to look after their own and their family's health. The information revolution is also about new ways of delivering care, such as enabling patients to communicate with their clinicians about their health status on-line. We will provide a range of on-line services which will mean services being provided much more efficiently at a time and place that is convenient for patients and carers, and will also enable greater efficiency.

2.7 Information generated by patients themselves will be critical to this process, and will include much wider use of effective tools like Patient-Reported Outcome Measures (PROMS), patient experience data, and real-time feedback. At present, PROMs, other outcome measures, patient experience surveys and national clinical audit are not used widely enough. We will expand their validity, collection and use. The Department will extend national clinical audit to support clinicians across a much wider range of treatments and conditions, and it will extend PROMs across the NHS wherever practicable.

2.8 We will also encourage more widespread use of patient experience surveys and real-time feedback. We will enable patients to rate services and clinical departments according to the quality of care they received, and we will require hospitals to be open about mistakes and always tell patients if something has gone wrong. We will also require that staff feedback around the quality of the patient care provided in organisations is publicly available. As in many other services, this feedback from patients, carers and families, and staff will help to inform other people with similar conditions to make the right choice of hospital or clinical department and will encourage providers to be more responsive.[21] The Department will seek views on how best to ensure this approach is developed in a coherent way.

2.9 Information will improve accountability: in future, it will be far easier for the public to see where unacceptable services are being provided and to exert local pressure for them to be improved. There is compelling evidence that better information also creates a clear drive for improvement in providers. Our intention is for clinical teams to see a meaningful, risk-adjusted assessment of their performance against their peers, and this assessment should also be placed in the public domain. The Department will revise and extend quality accounts to reinforce local accountability for performance, encourage peer competition, and provide a clear spur for boards of provider organisations to focus on improving outcomes. Subject to evaluation, we will extend quality accounts to all providers of NHS care from 2011 and continue to strengthen the independent assurance of quality accounts to ensure the content is accurate and fair. We will ensure that nationally comparable information is published, in a way that patients, their families and clinical teams can use.

2.10 More information about commissioning of healthcare will also improve public accountability. Wherever possible, we will ensure that information about services is published on a commissioner basis. We will also publish assessments of how well commissioners are performing, so that they are held to account for their use of public money.

> **Information to support choice and accountability**
>
> In future, there should be increasing amounts of robust information, comparable between similar providers, on:
>
> - **Safety**: for example, about levels of healthcare-associated infections, adverse events and avoidable deaths, broken down by providers and clinical teams;
>
> - **Effectiveness**: for example, mortality rates (this could include mortality from heart disease, and one year and five year cancer survival), emergency re-admission rates; and patient-reported outcome measures; and
>
> - **Experience**: including information on average and maximum waiting times; opening hours and clinic times; cancelled operations; and diverse measures of patient experience, based on feedback from patients, families and carers.

2.11   We will enable patients to have control of their health records. This will start with access to the records held by their GP and over time this will extend to health records held by all providers. The patient will determine who else can access their records and will easily be able to see changes when they are made to their records. We will consult on arrangements, including appropriate confidentiality safeguards, later this year.

2.12   Our aim is that people should be able to share their records with third parties, such as support groups for patients, who can help patients understand their records and manage their condition better. We will make it simple for a patient to download their record and pass it, in a standard format, to any organisation of their choice.

2.13   We intend to make aggregate data available in a standard format to allow intermediaries to analyse and present it to patients in an easily understandable way. Making aggregated, anonymised data available to the university and research sectors also has the potential to suggest new areas of research through medical and scientific analysis. There will be safeguards to protect personally identifiable information. We will consider introducing a voluntary accreditation system, which will allow information intermediaries to apply for a kitemark to demonstrate to the public that they meet quality standards.

2.14   Patients and carers will be able to access the information they want through a range of means, to ensure that no individual or section of the community is left out. In addition to NHS Choices, a range of third parties will be encouraged to provide information to support patient choice. Assistance will be provided for people who do not access on-line health advice, or who would particularly benefit from more intensive support.

2.15   We will ensure the right data is collected by the Health and Social Care Information Centre to enable people to exercise choice. We will seek to centralise all data returns in the Information Centre, which will have lead responsibility for data collection and assuring the data quality of those returns, working with other interested parties such as Monitor and the Care Quality Commission. We will also review data collections with a view to reducing burdens, as outlined in chapter 5. The forthcoming Health Bill will contain provisions to put the Information Centre on a firmer statutory footing, with clearer powers across organisations in the health and care system.

2.16   Providers will be under clear contractual obligations, with sanctions, in relation to accuracy and timeliness of data. Along with commissioners, they will have to use agreed technical and data standards to promote compatibility between different systems. The NHS Commissioning Board will determine these standards but they will include, for example, record keeping, data sharing capabilities, efficiency of data transfer and data security. We will clarify the legal ownership and responsibilities of organisations and people who manage health data. This may require primary legislation and we will consult on arrangements later this year.

2.17   The Department will publish an information strategy this autumn to seek views on how best to implement these changes.

Increased choice and control

2.18   In future, patients and carers will have far more clout and choice in the system; and as a result, the NHS will become more responsive to their needs and wishes. People want choice,[22] and evidence at home and abroad shows that it improves quality.[23] We are also clear that increasing patient choice is not a one-way street. In return for greater choice and control, patients should accept responsibility for the choices they make, concordance with treatment programmes and the implications for their lifestyle.

2.19   The previous Government made a start on patient choice, but its focus was narrow, concentrating mainly on choice of provider. Although limited progress has been made on choice of provider for first elective appointment, the policy has not been implemented fully and momentum has stalled. It has remained the case for several years that just under half of patients recall that their GP has offered them choice.[24] The Department will increase that significantly. We will explore with the profession and patient groups how we can make rapid progress towards this goal.

2.20   However, we do not see choice as just being about where you go and when, but a more fundamental control of the circumstances of the treatment and care you receive.

Extending choice

The Government will:

- Increase the current offer of **choice of any provider** significantly, and will explore with professional and patient groups how we can make rapid progress towards this goal;

- Create a presumption that all patients will have choice and control over their care and treatment, and **choice of any willing provider** wherever relevant (it will not be appropriate for all services – for example, emergency ambulance admissions to A&E);

- Introduce **choice of named consultant-led team** for elective care by April 2011 where clinically appropriate. We will look at ways of ensuring that Choose and Book usage is maximised, and we intend to amend the appropriate standard acute contract to ensure that providers list named consultants on Choose and Book;

- **Extend maternity choice** and help make safe, informed choices throughout pregnancy and in childbirth a reality – recognising that not all choices will be appropriate or safe for all women – by developing new provider networks. Pregnancy offers a unique opportunity to engage women from all sections of society, with the right support through pregnancy and at the start of life being vital for improving life chances and tackling cycles of disadvantage;

- Begin to introduce choice of treatment and provider in some **mental health services** from April 2011, and extend this wherever practicable;

- Begin to introduce choice for **diagnostic testing**, and **choice post-diagnosis**, from 2011;

- Introduce **choice in care for long-term conditions** as part of personalised care planning. In **end-of-life care**, we will move towards a national choice offer to support people's preferences about how to have a good death, and we will work with providers, including hospices, to ensure that people have the support they need;

- Give patients more information on **research studies** that are relevant to them, and more scope to join in if they wish;

- Give every patient a clear **right to choose to register with any GP practice** they want with an open list, without being restricted by where they live. People should be able to expect that they can change their GP quickly and straightforwardly if and when it is right for them, but

> equally that they can stay with their GP if they wish when they move house.
>
> - Develop **a coherent 24/7 urgent care service in every area of England** that makes sense to patients when they have to make choices about their care. This will incorporate GP out-of-hours services and provide urgent medical care for people registered with a GP elsewhere. We will make care more accessible by introducing, informed by evaluation, a single telephone number for every kind of urgent and social care and by using technology to help people communicate with their clinicians; and
>
> - Consult on **choice of treatment** later this year including the potential introduction of new contractual requirements.

2.21   In implementing proposals for extending choice, the Department will consult widely. We will need to tackle a range of issues, including: professional and patient engagement; reform to payment systems so that money follows the patient and enables choices to work; information availability and accessibility to enable choice of treatment, including decision aids, particularly in mental health and community services; support to patients with different language needs and patients with disabilities to ensure that they can exercise choice; ensuring that local commissioners fully support rather than restrict choice; and maximising use of Choose and Book. We will consult on choice of treatment later this year, including the potential introduction of new contractual requirements on providers, and collecting and publishing information on whether this is happening, to support patients.

2.22   The previous Government recently started a programme of personal health budget pilots. International evidence, and evidence from social care, shows that these have much potential to help improve outcomes, transform NHS culture by putting patients in control, and enable integration across health and social care. As part of personalised care planning, the Department will encourage further pilots to come forward and explore the potential for introducing a right to a personal health budget in discrete areas such as NHS continuing care. We also recognise that introducing personal budgets is operationally complex and the Government will use the results of the evaluation in 2012 to inform a wider, more general roll-out.

2.23   We expect choice of treatment and provider to become the reality for patients in the vast majority of NHS-funded services by no later than 2013/14. In future, the NHS Commissioning Board will have a key role in promoting and extending choice and control. It will be responsible for developing and agreeing with the Secretary of State guarantees for patients about the choices they can make, in order to provide clarity for patients and providers alike, ensuring the advice of Monitor is sought on any implications for competition. The Government will require the NHS Commissioning Board to develop an implementation plan as one of its first tasks, working with patient and professional groups; and the Secretary of State will hold it to account for progress.

Patient and public voice

2.24   We will strengthen the collective voice of patients, and we will bring forward provisions in the forthcoming Health Bill to create HealthWatch England, a new independent consumer champion within the Care Quality Commission. Local Involvement Networks (LINks) will become the local HealthWatch, creating a strong local infrastructure, and we will enhance the role of local authorities in promoting choice and complaints advocacy, through the HealthWatch arrangements they commission.

2.25   We will also look at existing mechanisms, including relevant legislation, to ensure that public engagement is fully effective in future, and that services meet the needs of neighbourhoods.

2.26   All sources of feedback, of which complaints are an important part, should be a central mechanism for providers to assess the quality of their services. We want to avoid the experience of Mid-Staffordshire, where patient and staff concerns were continually overlooked while systemic failure in the quality of care went unchecked. Building on existing complaints handling structures, we will strengthen arrangements for information sharing. Local HealthWatch will also have the power to recommend that poor services are investigated.

The role of HealthWatch

At local level:

- Local HealthWatch organisations will ensure that the views and feedback from patients and carers are an integral part of local commissioning across health and social care;

- Local authorities will be able to commission local HealthWatch or HealthWatch England to provide advocacy and support, helping people access and make choices about services, and supporting individuals who want to make a complaint. In particular, they will support people who lack the means or capacity to make choices; for example, helping them choose which General Practice to register with;

- Local HealthWatch will be funded by and accountable to local authorities, and will be involved in local authorities' new partnership functions, described in chapter 4. To reinforce local accountability, local authorities will be responsible for ensuring that local HealthWatch are operating

---

effectively, and for putting in place better arrangements if they are not; and

- Local HealthWatch will provide a source of intelligence for national HealthWatch and will be able to report concerns about the quality of providers, independently of the local authority.

At national level:

- HealthWatch England will provide leadership, advice and support to local HealthWatch, and will be able to provide advocacy services on their behalf if the local authority wishes;

- HealthWatch England will provide advice to the Health and Social Care Information Centre on the information which would be of most use to patients to facilitate their choices about their care;

- HealthWatch England will provide advice to the NHS Commissioning Board, Monitor and the Secretary of State; and

- Based on information received from local HealthWatch and other sources, HealthWatch England will have powers to propose CQC investigations of poor services.

Figure 1

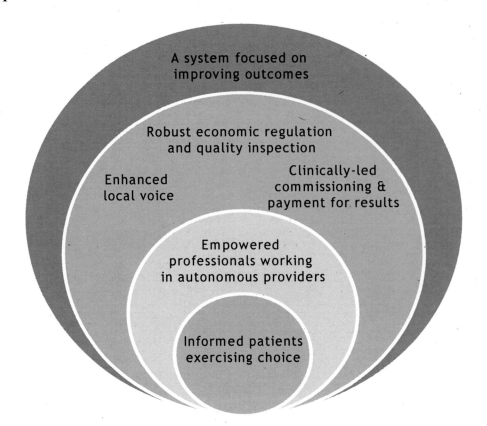

3.   Improving healthcare outcomes

3.1   The primary purpose of the NHS is to improve the outcomes of healthcare for all: to deliver care that is safer, more effective, and that provides a better experience for patients. Building on Lord Darzi's work, the Government will now establish improvement in quality and healthcare outcomes as the primary purpose of all NHS-funded care. This primary purpose will be enshrined in statute, the NHS Constitution, and model contracts for services, ensuring that the focus is always on what matters most to patients and professionals.

3.2   We will start by discarding what blocks progress in the NHS today: the overwhelming importance attached to certain top-down targets. These targets crowd out the bigger objectives of reducing mortality and morbidity, increasing safety and improving patient experience more broadly – including for the most vulnerable in our society. We have already revised the NHS Operating Framework for 2010/11, setting out how existing targets should be treated this year. Some targets are clinically justifiable and deliver significant benefits. Others, that have no clinical relevance, have been removed. In future, performance will be driven by patient choice and commissioning; as a result, there will be no excuse or hiding place for deteriorating standards and our proposals will drive improving standards.

3.3   This will help ensure that patient safety is placed above all else at the heart of the NHS, and that there are no longer any production line approaches to healthcare, which measure the volume but ignore the quality. There cannot be a trade-off between safety and efficiency. Our information revolution will play an important role in this, boosting transparency so that failings do not go undetected. It will help foster a culture of active responsibility where staff and patients are empowered to ask, challenge and intervene.

3.4   We will replace the relationship between politicians and professionals with relationships between professionals and patients. Instead of national process targets, the NHS will, wherever possible, use clinically credible and evidence-based measures that clinicians themselves use. The Government believes that outcomes will improve most rapidly when clinicians are engaged, and creativity, research participation and professionalism are allowed to flourish. In future, the Secretary of State will hold the NHS to account for improving healthcare outcomes. The NHS, not politicians, will be responsible for determining how best to deliver this within a clear and coherent national policy framework.

The NHS Outcomes Framework

3.5 The current performance regime will be replaced with separate frameworks for outcomes that set direction for the NHS, for public health and social care, which provide for clear and unambiguous accountability, and enable better joint working. The Secretary of State, through the Public Health Service, will set local authorities national objectives for improving population health outcomes. It will be for local authorities to determine how best to secure those objectives, including by commissioning services from providers of NHS care.

3.6 A new NHS Outcomes Framework will provide direction for the NHS. It will include a focused set of national outcome goals determined by the Secretary of State, against which the NHS Commissioning Board will be held to account, alongside overall improvements in the NHS.

3.7 In turn, the NHS Outcomes Framework will be translated into a commissioning outcomes framework for GP consortia, to create powerful incentives for effective commissioning.

3.8 The NHS Outcomes Framework will span the three domains of quality:

- the effectiveness of the treatment and care provided to patients – measured by both clinical outcomes and patient-reported outcomes;

- the safety of the treatment and care provided to patients; and

- the broader experience patients have of the treatment and care they receive.

For example, effectiveness goals might include how we compare internationally on avoidable mortality and morbidity across a range of conditions. The criteria used will ensure that we do not exclude outcomes for key groups and services such as children, older people and mental health.

3.9 The Department will launch a consultation on the development of the national outcome goals. We are committed to working with clinicians, patients, carers and representative groups to create indicators that are based on the best available evidence. Later this year, in the light of the Spending Review, the Government will issue the first NHS Outcomes Framework. We intend it will be available to support NHS organisations in delivering improved outcomes from April 2011, with full implementation from April 2012.

3.10 The NHS Commissioning Board will work with clinicians, patients and the public at every level of the system to develop the NHS Outcomes Framework into a more comprehensive set of indicators, reflecting the quality standards developed by NICE. The framework and its constituent indicators will enable international comparisons wherever possible, and reflect the Board's duties to promote equality and tackle inequalities in healthcare outcomes. It will ensure that clinical values direct managerial activity and that every part of the NHS is focusing on the right goals for patients. The main purpose of the programme of reform set out in this White Paper is to change the NHS environment so that it is easier to progress against those goals.

3.11 It is essential for patient outcomes that health and social care services are better integrated at all levels of the system. We will be consulting widely on options to ensure health and social care works seamlessly together to enable this.

Developing and implementing quality standards

3.12 Progress on outcomes will be supported by quality standards. These will be developed for the NHS Commissioning Board by NICE, who will develop authoritative standards setting out each part of the patient pathway, and indicators for each step. NICE will rapidly expand its existing work programme to create a comprehensive library of standards for all the main pathways of care. The first three on stroke, dementia and prevention of venous thromboembolism were published in June. Within the next five years, NICE expects to produce 150 standards. To support the development of quality standards, NICE will advise the National Institute for Health Research on research priorities.

3.13 Each standard is a set of 5-10 specific, concise quality statements and associated measures. These measures act as markers of high quality, cost-effective patient care. They are about excellence, derived from the best available evidence and are produced collaboratively with the NHS and social care professionals, along with their partners, service users and carers. The standards will be developed in a way that makes sense for patients, and they will extend beyond NHS care, informing the work of local authorities and the Public Health Service. They will include information for clinicians and patients on relevant and ongoing research studies that are key to improving evidence for better outcomes.

3.14 With the increasing importance of coherent joint arrangements between health and social care, the standards will cover areas that span health and social care. We will expand the role of NICE to develop quality standards for social care. The Health Bill will put NICE on a firmer statutory footing, securing its independence and core functions and extending its remit to social care.

NICE quality standard for venous thromboembolism (VTE)

Quality statements:

- All patients, on admission, receive an assessment of VTE and bleeding risk using the clinical risk assessment criteria described in the national tool.

- Patients/carers are offered verbal and written information on VTE prevention

---

as part of the admission process.

- Patients provided with anti-embolism stockings have them fitted and monitored in accordance with NICE guidance.

- Patients are re-assessed within 24 hours of admission for risk of VTE and bleeding.

- Patients assessed to be at risk of VTE are offered VTE prophylaxis in accordance with NICE guidance.

- Patients/carers are offered verbal and written information on VTE prevention as part of the discharge process.

- Patients are offered extended (post-hospital) VTE prophylaxis in accordance with NICE guidance.[25]

3.15   Commissioners will draw from the NICE library of standards as they commission care. GP consortia and providers will agree local priorities for implementation each year, taking account of the NHS Outcomes Framework. NICE quality standards will be reflected in commissioning contracts and financial incentives. Together with essential regulatory standards, these will provide the national consistency that patients expect from their National Health Service.

Research

3.16   The Government is committed to the promotion and conduct of research as a core NHS role. Research is vital in providing the new knowledge needed to improve health outcomes and reduce inequalities. Research is even more important when resources are under pressure – it identifies new ways of preventing, diagnosing and treating disease. It is essential if we are to increase the quality and productivity of the NHS, and to support growth in the economy. A thriving life sciences industry is critical to the ability of the NHS to deliver world-class health outcomes. The Department will continue to promote the role of Biomedical Research Centres and Units, Academic Health Science Centres and Collaborations for Leadership in Applied Health Research and Care, to develop research and to unlock synergies between research, education and patient care.

Incentives for quality improvement

3.17   The absence of an effective payment system in many parts of the NHS severely restricts the ability of commissioners and providers to improve outcomes, increase efficiency and increase patient choice. In future, the structure of payment systems will be the responsibility of the NHS Commissioning Board, and the economic regulator will be responsible for pricing. In the meantime the Department will start designing and implementing a more comprehensive, transparent and sustainable structure of payment for performance so that money follows the patient and reflects quality. Payments and the 'currencies' they are based on will be structured in the way that is most relevant to the service being provided, and will be conditional on achieving quality goals.

3.18 The previous administration made progress in developing payment by results in acute trusts. The mandatory scope has changed little since 2005/06, and has not incentivised results throughout the system. The Department will:

- implement a set of currencies for adult mental health services for use from 2012/13, and develop currencies for child and adolescent services;

- develop payment systems to support the commissioning of talking therapies;

- mandate in 2011/12 national currencies for adult and neonatal critical care;

- review payment systems to support end-of-life care, including exploring options for per-patient funding;

- accelerate the development of pathway tariffs for use by commissioners;

- accelerate the development of currencies and tariffs for community services;

- implement in 2011/12 further incentives to reduce avoidable readmissions and encourage more joined-up working between hospitals and social care for services following discharge; and

- link quality measures in national clinical audits to payment arrangements.

3.19 The Department will also refine the basis of current tariffs. We will rapidly accelerate the development of best-practice tariffs, introducing an increasing number each year, so that providers are paid according to the costs of excellent care, rather than average price. 2011/12 will see the introduction of best-practice tariffs for interventional radiology, day-case surgery for breast surgery, hernia repairs and some orthopaedic surgery. The Department will also introduce the latest version of the International Classification of Disease (ICD) 10 clinical diagnosis coding system from 2012/13, and explore the scope for developing a benchmarking approach, with greater local flexibility, including for local marginal rates.

3.20 If providers deliver excellent care in line with commissioner priorities, the commissioner will be able to pay a quality increment. The Department will extend the scope and value of the Commissioning for Quality and Innovation (CQUIN) payment framework, to support local quality improvement goals. The CQUIN framework will be important for the implementation of NICE quality standards and improving patient experience and patient-reported outcomes. And in future, if providers deliver poor quality care, the commissioner will also be able to impose a contractual penalty. In particular, we will proceed with work to impose fines for an extended list of "never events", such as wrong site surgery, from October 2010.[26]

3.21   The principle of rewarding quality will also apply in primary care. In general practice the Department will seek over time to establish a single contractual and funding model to promote quality improvement, deliver fairness for all practices, support free patient choice, and remove unnecessary barriers to new provision. Our principle is that funding should follow the registered patient, on a weighted capitation model, adjusted for quality. We will incentivise ways of improving access to primary care in disadvantaged areas.

3.22   Following consultation and piloting, we will introduce a new dentistry contract, with a focus on improving quality, achieving good dental health and increasing access to NHS dentistry, and an additional focus on the oral health of schoolchildren. The community pharmacy contract, through payment for performance, will incentivise and support high quality and efficient services, including better value in the use of medicines through better informed and more involved patients. Pharmacists, working with doctors and other health professionals, have an important and expanding role in optimising the use of medicines and in supporting better health. Pharmacy services will benefit from greater transparency in NHS pricing and payment for services.

3.23   The Government will also reform the way that drug companies are paid for NHS medicines, moving to a system of value-based pricing when the current scheme expires. This will help ensure better access for patients to effective drugs and innovative treatments on the NHS and secure value for money for NHS spending on medicines. As an interim measure, the Department is creating a new Cancer Drug Fund, which will operate from April 2011; this fund will help patients get the cancer drugs their doctors recommend.

4. Autonomy, accountability and democratic legitimacy

4.1   The Government's reforms will liberate professionals and providers from top-down control. This is the only way to secure the quality, innovation and productivity needed to improve outcomes. We will give responsibility for commissioning and budgets to groups of GP practices; and providers will be freed from government control to shape their services around the needs and choices of patients. Greater autonomy will be matched by increased accountability to patients and democratic legitimacy, with a transparent regime of economic regulation and quality inspection to hold providers to account for the results they deliver.

GP commissioning consortia

4.2   In order to shift decision-making as close as possible to individual patients, the Department will devolve power and responsibility for commissioning services to local consortia of GP practices. This change will build on the pivotal and trusted role that primary care professionals already play in coordinating patient care, through the system of registered patient lists.

4.3   Primary care professionals coordinate all the services that patients receive, helping them to navigate the system and ensure they get the best care (of course, they do not deliver all the care themselves). For this reason they are best placed to coordinate the commissioning of care for their patients while involving all other clinical professionals who are also part of any pathway of care.

4.4   Commissioning by GP consortia will mean that the redesign of patient pathways and local services is always clinically-led and based on more effective dialogue and partnership with hospital specialists. It will bring together responsibility for clinical decisions and for the financial consequences of these decisions. This will reinforce the crucial role that GPs already play in committing NHS resources through their daily clinical decisions – not only in terms of referrals and prescribing, but also how well they manage long-term conditions, and the accessibility of their services. It will increase efficiency, by enabling GPs to strip out activities that do not have appreciable benefits for patients' health or healthcare.

4.5   GP-led purchasing has history. Practice-based commissioning was an attempt by the last Government to build on the successful parts of previous Conservative approaches, such as total purchasing pilots. There have been some examples of practice-based groups making progress, in spite of a flawed policy framework that confuses the respective responsibilities of GPs and PCTs, and fails to transfer real freedom and responsibility to GP practices. Our model is neither a recreation of GP fundholding nor a complete rejection of practice-based commissioning. Fundholding led to a two-tier NHS; and practice-based commissioning never became a real transfer of responsibility. So we will learn from the past, and offer a clear way forward for GP consortia.

4.6 The Government will shortly issue a document setting out our proposals in more detail, and providing the basis for fuller engagement with primary care professionals, patients and the public. We will then bring forward legislation in the forthcoming Health Bill.

The role of GP commissioning consortia

- We envisage putting GP commissioning on a statutory basis, with powers and duties set out in primary and secondary legislation.

- Consortia of GP practices, working with other health and care professionals, and in partnership with local communities and local authorities, will commission the great majority of NHS services for their patients. They will not be directly responsible for commissioning services that GPs themselves provide, but they will become increasingly influential in driving up the quality of general practice. They will not commission the other family health services of dentistry, community pharmacy and primary ophthalmic services. These will be the responsibility of the NHS Commissioning Board, as will national and regional specialised services, although consortia will have influence and involvement.

- The NHS Commissioning Board will calculate practice-level budgets and allocate these directly to consortia. The consortia will hold contracts with providers and may choose to adopt a lead commissioner model, for example in relation to large teaching hospitals.

- GP consortia will include an accountable officer, and the NHS Commissioning Board will be responsible for holding consortia to account for stewardship of NHS resources and for the outcomes they achieve as commissioners. In turn, each consortium will hold its constituent practices to account against these objectives.

- A fundamental principle of the new arrangements is that every GP practice will be a member of a consortium, as a corollary of holding a registered list of patients. Practices will have flexibility within the new legislative framework to form consortia in ways that they think will secure the best healthcare and health outcomes for their patients and locality. We envisage that the NHS Commissioning Board will be under a duty to establish a comprehensive system of GP consortia, and we

---

envisage a reserve power for the NHS Commissioning Board to be able to assign practices to consortia if necessary.

- GP consortia will need to have a sufficient geographic focus to be able to take responsibility for agreeing and monitoring contracts for locality-based services (such as urgent care services), to have responsibility for commissioning services for people who are not registered with a GP practice, and to commission services jointly with local authorities. The consortia will also need to be of sufficient size to manage financial risk and allow for accurate allocations.

- GP consortia will be responsible for managing the combined commissioning budgets of their member GP practices, and using these resources to improve healthcare and health outcomes. The Government will discuss with the BMA and the profession how primary medical care contracts can best reflect new complementary responsibilities for individual GP practices, including being a member of a consortium and supporting the consortium in ensuring efficient and effective use of NHS resources.

- GP consortia will need to have sufficient freedoms to use resources in ways that achieve the best and most cost-efficient outcomes for patients. Monitor and the NHS Commissioning Board will ensure that commissioning decisions are fair and transparent, and will promote competition.

- GP consortia will have the freedom to decide what commissioning activities they undertake for themselves and for what activities (such as demographic analysis, contract negotiation, performance monitoring and aspects of financial management) they may choose to buy in support from external organisations, including local authorities, private and voluntary sector bodies.

- We envisage that consortia will receive a maximum management allowance to reflect the costs associated with commissioning, with a premium for achieving high quality outcomes and for financial performance.

- GP consortia will have a duty to promote equalities and to work in partnership with local authorities, for instance in relation to health and adult social care, early years services, public health, safeguarding, and the wellbeing of local populations.

- GP consortia will have a duty of public and patient involvement, and will need to engage patients and the public in their neighbourhoods in the commissioning process. Through its local infrastructure, HealthWatch

> will provide evidence about local communities and their needs and aspirations.

4.7   A number of PCTs have made important progress in developing commissioning experience which we will be looking to capitalise on during the transition period. Through the transitional arrangements, we will seek to ensure that existing expertise and capability in primary care trusts (PCTs) is maintained during the transition period where this is the wish of GP consortia.

4.8   Primary care trusts will have an important task in the next two years in supporting practices to prepare for these new arrangements. We want implementation to be driven bottom-up, with GP consortia taking on their new responsibilities as rapidly as possible, and early adopters promoting best practice.

4.9   The final shape of these proposals will depend upon our consultation findings and developing clear arrangements for managing financial risk. Our indicative timetable is for:

- a comprehensive system of GP consortia in place in shadow form during 2011/12, taking on increased delegated responsibility from PCTs;

- following passage of the Health Bill, consortia to take on responsibility for commissioning in 2012/13;

- the NHS Commissioning Board to make allocations for 2013/14 directly to GP consortia in late 2012; and

- GP consortia to take full financial responsibility from April 2013.

An autonomous NHS Commissioning Board

4.10   To support GP consortia in their commissioning decisions we will create a statutory NHS Commissioning Board. This will be a lean and expert organisation, free from day-to-day political interference, with a commissioning model that draws from best international practice. The NHS Commissioning Board will provide leadership for quality improvement through commissioning: through commissioning guidelines, it will help standardise what is known good practice, for example improving discharge from hospital, maximising the number of day care operations, reducing delays prior to operations, and enabling community access to care and treatments. It will play its full part in promoting equality in line with the Equality Act 2010. It will not manage providers or be the NHS headquarters.

4.11   The Board will promote patient and carer involvement and choice, championing the interests of the patient rather than the interests of particular providers. It will involve patients as a matter of course in its business, for example in developing commissioning guidelines. To avoid double jeopardy and duplication, it will take over the current CQC responsibility of assessing NHS commissioners and will hold GP consortia to account for their performance and quality. It will manage some national and regional commissioning. It will allocate and account for NHS resources. It will have a role in supporting the Secretary of State and the Public Health Service to ensure that the NHS in England is resilient and able to be mobilised during any emergency it faces, or as part of a national response to threats external to the NHS. It will promote involvement in research and the use of research evidence.

The role of the NHS Commissioning Board

The Board will have five main functions:

1. **Providing national leadership on commissioning for quality improvement:**

   - setting commissioning guidelines on the basis of clinically approved quality standards developed with the advice of NICE in a way that promotes joint working across health, public health and social care;

   - designing model contracts for local commissioners to adapt and use with providers;

   - designing the structure of tariff and other financial incentives, whilst Monitor will set tariff levels;

   - hosting some clinical commissioning networks, for example for rarer cancers and transplant services, to pool specialist expertise;

   - setting standards for the quality of NHS commissioning and procurement;

   - making available accessible information on commissioner performance; and

   - tackling inequalities in outcomes of healthcare.

2. **Promoting and extending public and patient involvement and choice:**

   - championing greater involvement of patients and carers in decision-making and managing their own care, working with commissioners and local authorities;

   - promoting personalisation and extending patient choice of what, where and who, including personal health budgets; and

   - commissioning information requirements for choice and for

accountability, including through patient-reported measures.

3. **Ensuring the development of GP commissioning consortia:**

   - supporting and developing the establishment and maintenance of an effective and comprehensive system of GP consortia; and

   - holding consortia to account for delivering outcomes and financial performance.

4. **Commissioning certain services** that cannot solely be commissioned by consortia, in accordance with Secretary of State designation, including:

   - GP, dentistry, community pharmacy and primary ophthalmic services;

   - national specialised services[27] and regional specialised services set out in the Specialised Services National Definitions Set;[28] and

   - maternity services.

5. **Allocating and accounting for NHS resources:**

   - allocating NHS revenue resources to GP consortia on the basis of seeking to secure equivalent access to NHS services relative to the burden of disease and disability;

   - managing an overall NHS commissioner revenue limit, for which it will be accountable to the Department of Health; and

   - promoting productivity through better commissioning.

The Board would not have the power to restrict the scope of the services offered by the NHS.

Establishing the Board and managing the transition

4.12   The Board will be established in shadow form as a special health authority from April 2011. In 2011/12 it will develop its future business model, organisational structure and staffing. It will be converted by the forthcoming Health Bill into a statutory body, with its own powers and duties, and will go live in April 2012.

4.13   Changes in the way that strategic health authorities (SHA) operate will help pave the way for the NHS Commissioning Board. From this year SHAs will separate their commissioning and provider oversight functions. They will support the Board during its preparatory year, and have a critical role during the transition in managing finance and performance. It will be for the NHS Commissioning Board to decide what, if any, presence it needs in different parts of the country. SHAs will be abolished as statutory bodies during 2012/13. From 2012 the Board will perform those national functions relevant to its new role that are currently carried out by the Department of Health. It will be subject to clear controls over management costs and consultancy spend.

A new relationship between the NHS and the Government

4.14 At present the Secretary of State enjoys extraordinarily wide powers over the NHS. It is intended that the forthcoming Health Bill will introduce provisions to limit the ability of the Secretary of State to micromanage and intervene. The forthcoming Health Bill will formalise the relationship between the government and the NHS, to improve transparency and increase stability, while maintaining the necessary level of political accountability for such large amounts of taxpayers' money.

The NHS role of the Secretary of State

The key NHS-related functions of the Secretary of State will include:

- **Setting a formal mandate for the NHS Commissioning Board.** This will be subject to consultation and Parliamentary scrutiny, and will include specific levels of improvement against a small number of outcome indicators.

- **Holding the NHS Commissioning Board to account.** In addition to delivery of improvements against the agreed outcome indicators, the Secretary of State will hold the Board to account on delivering improvements in choice and patient involvement, and in maintaining financial control. Clear financial controls and associated financial instructions will be set by the Secretary of State in line with the Department's continued Parliamentary accountability for expenditure and HM Treasury requirements.

- **Arbitration.** The Secretary of State will have a statutory role as arbiter of last resort in disputes that arise between NHS commissioners and local authorities, for example in relation to major service changes.

- **The legislative and policy framework.** Responsibility for Department of State functions will remain with the Secretary of State. This includes determining the comprehensive service which the NHS provides, and developing and publishing national service strategies which will enable the roles of NHS, public health services and social care services to be better coordinated.

> - **Accounting annually to Parliament** for the overall performance of the NHS, public health and social care systems.

4.15 In future, the Secretary of State will be obliged to lay out a short formal mandate for the NHS Commissioning Board. This will be subject to public consultation and Parliamentary scrutiny, including by the Health Select Committee. The mandate is likely to be over a three year period, updated annually. The mandate will set out the totality of what the Government expects from the NHS Commissioning Board on behalf of the taxpayer for that period. This will comprise progress against outcomes specified by the Secretary of State, and objectives in relation to its core functions. Should the Government wish, by exception, to impose additional performance requirements on the Board in-year, it will on each occasion be obliged to lay a report in Parliament to explain why. The Secretary of State will also lose existing powers to intervene in relation to any specific commissioner other than in discharging defined statutory responsibilities. To ensure transparency, a public record will be made of all meetings between the Board and the Secretary of State.

Local democratic legitimacy

4.16 Following the establishment of the NHS Commissioning Board and a comprehensive network of GP consortia, PCTs will no longer have NHS commissioning functions. To realise administrative cost savings, and achieve greater alignment with local government responsibilities for local health and wellbeing, the Government will transfer PCT health improvement functions to local authorities and abolish PCTs. We expect that PCTs will cease to exist from 2013, in light of the successful establishment of GP consortia. Local Directors of Public Health will be jointly appointed by local authorities and the Public Health Service. Local Directors of Public Health will also have statutory duties in respect of the Public Health Service.

4.17 The Government will strengthen the local democratic legitimacy of the NHS. Building on the power of the local authority to promote local wellbeing, we will establish new statutory arrangements within local authorities – which will be established as "health and wellbeing boards" or within existing strategic partnerships – to take on the function of joining up the commissioning of local NHS services, social care and health improvement. These health and wellbeing boards allow local authorities to take a strategic approach and promote integration across health and adult social care, children's services, including safeguarding, and the wider local authority agenda.

4.18 We will simplify and extend the use of powers that enable joint working between the NHS and local authorities. It will be easier for commissioners and providers to adopt partnership arrangements, and adapt them to local circumstances.

4.19   These arrangements will give local authorities influence over NHS commissioning, and corresponding influence for NHS commissioners in relation to public health and social care. While NHS commissioning will be the sole preserve of the NHS Commissioning Board and GP consortia, our aim is to ensure coherent and coordinated local commissioning strategies across all three services, for example in relation to mental health or elderly care. The Secretary of State will seek to ensure strategic coordination nationally; the local authority's new functions will enable strategic coordination locally. It will not involve day-to-day interventions in NHS services. The Government will consult fully on the details of the new arrangements.

Local authorities' new functions

Each local authority will take on the function of joining up the commissioning of local NHS services, social care and health improvement.

Local authorities will therefore be responsible for:

- Promoting **integration and partnership working** between the NHS, social care, public health and other local services and strategies;

- Leading **joint strategic needs assessments**, and promoting collaboration on local commissioning plans, including by supporting joint commissioning arrangements where each party so wishes; and

- Building partnership for **service changes and priorities**. There will be an escalation process to the NHS Commissioning Board and the Secretary of State, which retain accountability for NHS commissioning decisions.

These functions would replace the current statutory functions of Health Overview and Scrutiny Committees.

As well as elected members of the local authority, all relevant NHS commissioners will be involved in carrying out these functions, as will the Directors of Public Health, adult social services, and children's services. They will all be under duties of partnership. Local HealthWatch representatives will also play a formal role to ensure that feedback from patients and service users is reflected in commissioning plans.

Freeing existing NHS providers

4.20   Autonomy in commissioning will be matched by autonomy for providers. Previous governments have tried to give greater freedom to providers, most recently through the introduction of foundation trusts. Yet the policy was flawed from the outset by the controls imposed upon foundation trusts by Whitehall. Meanwhile, the drive to extend foundation status across the NHS has lost momentum, leaving reform half completed.

4.21   Our ambition is to create the largest and most vibrant social enterprise sector in the world. The Government's intention is to free foundation trusts from constraints they are under, in line with their original conception, so they can innovate to improve care for patients. In future, they will be regulated in the same way as any other providers, whether from the private or voluntary sector. Patients will be able to choose care from the provider they think to be the best. As all NHS trusts become foundation trusts, staff will have an opportunity to transform their organisations into employee-led social enterprises that they themselves control, freeing them to use their front-line experience to structure services around what works best for patients. For many foundation trusts, a governance model involving staff, the public and patients works well but we recognise that this may not be the best model for all types of foundation trust, particularly smaller organisations such as those providing community services. We will consult on future requirements: we envisage that some foundation trusts will be led only by employees; others will have wider memberships. The benefits of this approach will be seen in high productivity, greater innovation, better care and greater job satisfaction. Foundation trusts will not be privatised.

4.22   Ahead of bringing forward legislation, we intend to consult on options for increasing foundation trusts' freedoms – while ensuring financial risk is properly managed – including:

- abolishing the arbitrary cap on the amount of income foundation trusts may earn from other sources to reinvest in their services and allowing a broader scope, for example to provide health and care services;

- enabling foundation trusts to merge more easily; and

- whether we should enable foundation trusts to tailor their governance arrangements to their local needs, within a broad statutory framework that ensures any surplus and any proceeds are reinvested in the organisation rather than distributed externally.

4.23   Within three years, we will support all NHS trusts to become foundation trusts. It will not be an option for organisations to decide to remain as an NHS trust rather than become or be part of a foundation trust and in due course, we will repeal the NHS trust legislative model. A new unit in the Department of Health will drive progress and oversee SHAs' responsibilities in relation to providers. In the event that a few NHS trusts and SHAs fail to agree credible plans, and where the NHS trust is unsustainable, the Secretary of State may as a matter of last resort apply the trust administration regime set out in the Health Act 2009.[29] From April 2013, Monitor will take on the responsibility of regulating all providers of NHS care, irrespective of their status. Financial control will be maintained during the transition, with the Department, Monitor and SHAs taking any necessary steps.

4.24 The Government will apply a consistent approach across all types of NHS services. We will end the uncertainty and delay about the future of community health services currently provided within PCTs. We will complete the separation of commissioning from provision by April 2011 and move as soon as possible to an "any willing provider" approach for community services, reducing barriers to entry by new suppliers. In future, all community services will be provided by foundation trusts or other types of provider.

4.25 Special statutory arrangements will be made for the three high secure psychiatric hospitals (Broadmoor, Rampton and Ashworth), allowing them to benefit from the independence of foundation status while retaining appropriate safeguards to reflect their role in the criminal justice system.

Economic regulation and quality inspection to enable provider freedom

4.26 Providers will no longer be part of a system of top-down management, subject to political interference. Instead, they will be governed by a stable, transparent and rules-based system of regulation. Our aim is to free up provision of healthcare, so that in most sectors of care, any willing provider can provide services, giving patients greater choice and ensuring effective competition stimulates innovation and improvements, and increases productivity within a social market.

4.27 As now, the Care Quality Commission will act as quality inspectorate across health and social care for both publicly and privately funded care. In addition, we will develop Monitor, the current independent regulator of foundation trusts, into an economic regulator from April 2012, with responsibility for all providers of NHS care from April 2013. Providers will have a joint licence overseen by both Monitor and CQC, to maintain essential levels of safety and quality and ensure continuity of essential services.

The role of the Care Quality Commission

We will strengthen the role of CQC as an effective quality inspectorate by giving it a clearer focus on the essential levels of safety and quality of providers. In relation to the NHS, CQC's responsibilities will include:

Licensing - Together with Monitor, CQC will operate a joint licensing regime, with CQC being responsible for licensing against the essential safety and quality requirements. Where services fail to meet these essential levels, providers will be subject to enforcement action, including the possibility of fines and suspension of services.

Inspections - CQC will inspect providers against the essential levels of safety and quality. Inspection will be targeted and risk-based. CQC will carry out

---

inspections of providers in response to information that it receives about a provider. This information will come through a range of sources including patient feedback and complaints, HealthWatch, GP consortia and the NHS Commissioning Board. Where inspection reveals that a provider is not meeting essential levels of safety and quality, CQC will take enforcement action to bring about improvement.

The role of Monitor

Monitor will be turned into the economic regulator for the health and social care sectors, with three key functions:

- **Promoting competition**, to ensure that competition works effectively in the interests of patients and taxpayers. Like other sectoral regulators, such as OFCOM and OFGEM, Monitor will have concurrent powers with the Office of Fair Trading to apply competition law[30] to prevent anti-competitive behaviour;

- **Price regulation**. Where price regulation is necessary, Monitor's role will be to set efficient prices, or maximum prices, for NHS-funded services, in order to promote fair competition and drive productivity. In setting prices, Monitor will be required to consult the NHS Commissioning Board and take account of patients and taxpayers' interests including the need to secure the most efficient use of available resources; and

- **Supporting continuity of services**. Primary responsibility for ensuring continuity of services will lie with the NHS Commissioning Board and local commissioners. However, Monitor will also play a role in ensuring continued access to key services in some cases. Monitor will be responsible for defining regulated services that will be subject to special licence conditions and controls.

Monitor's levers to ensure that essential services are maintained will include:

- powers to protect assets or facilities required to maintain continuity of essential services;

- authorising special funding arrangements for essential services that would otherwise be unviable (with the agreement of the NHS Commissioning Board, and subject to rules on state aid);

- powers to levy providers for contributions to a risk pool; and

> • intervening directly in the event of failure, including power to trigger a special administration and regime.

Monitor's scope and powers

4.28 Like other sectoral regulators, we propose that Monitor should have proactive, "*ex ante*" powers to protect essential services and help open the NHS social market up to competition, as well as being able to take "*ex post*" enforcement action reactively. *Ex ante* powers would enable Monitor, for instance, to protect essential assets; require monopoly providers to grant access to their facilities to third parties; or conduct market studies and refer potential structural problems to the Competition Commission for investigation. To minimise the risks of excessive regulation, the need for *ex ante* powers would be reviewed over time. In most regulated industries, the focus of competition regulation is on preventing anti-competitive behaviour by powerful suppliers. However, within the NHS social market, there is also scope for purchasers to act anti-competitively, for example by failing to tender services or discriminating in favour of incumbent providers. Monitor will be able to investigate complaints of anti-competitive purchasing and act as arbiter.

4.29 Monitor's powers to regulate prices and license providers will only cover publicly-funded health services. However, its powers to apply competition law will extend to both publicly and privately funded healthcare, and to social care.

4.30 The Government will shortly issue a document setting out our proposals on foundation trusts and economic regulation in more detail, for consultation, prior to bringing forward provisions in the forthcoming Health Bill.

Figure 2

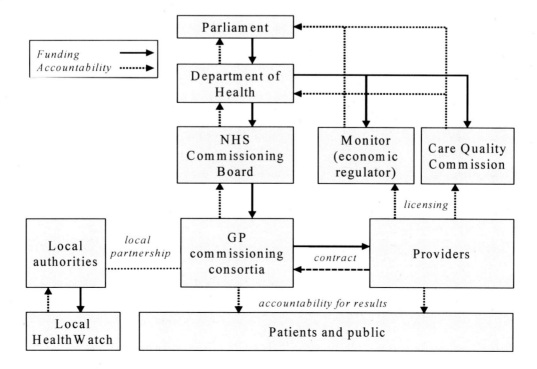

39

Valuing staff

4.31   Staff who are empowered, engaged and well supported provide better patient care. We will therefore promote staff engagement, partnership working and the implementation of Dr Steve Boorman's recommendations to improve staff health and wellbeing.[31] We will also extend the principles of autonomy, not only by giving professionals more control of the way that NHS services are commissioned and provided, but also in our approach to staff training, education and pay.

Training and education

4.32   Each year several billion pounds are spent on central funding of education and training for NHS staff through the Multi-Profession Education and Training levy, in addition to investment by NHS organisations in their own staff. A top-down management approach led by the Department of Health does not allow accountability for decisions affecting workforce supply and demand to sit in the right place. It is time to give employers greater autonomy and accountability for planning and developing the workforce, alongside greater professional ownership of the quality of education and training.

4.33   In future, the Department will have a progressively reducing role in overseeing education and training. The system will be designed to ensure that education and training commissioning is aligned locally and nationally with the commissioning of patient care. Our vision is that:

- Healthcare employers and their staff will agree plans and funding for workforce development and training; their decisions will determine education commissioning plans.

- Education commissioning will be led locally and nationally by the healthcare professions, through Medical Education England for doctors, dentists, healthcare scientists and pharmacists. Similar mechanisms will be put in place for nurses and midwives and the allied health professions. They will work with employers to ensure a multi-disciplinary approach that meets their local needs.

- The professions will have a leading role in deciding the structure and content of training, and quality standards.

- All providers of healthcare services will pay to meet the costs of education and training. Transparent funding flows for education and training will support the level playing field between providers.

- The NHS Commissioning Board will provide national patient and public

> oversight of healthcare providers' funding plans for training and education, checking that these reflect its strategic commissioning intentions. GP consortia will provide this oversight at local level.
>
> - The Centre for Workforce Intelligence will act as a consistent source of information and analysis, informing and informed by all levels of the system.

4.34 The Department will publish proposals for consultation in due course. Reforms will be managed and introduced carefully to ensure that the changes do not de-stabilise individual providers.

NHS pay

4.35 Ministers currently exercise substantial control over pay levels and contractual arrangements for NHS staff. In the short term, the need for fiscal consolidation is paramount and this will require sustained pay restraint across the public sector. The NHS must play its part as the largest public service in the country. We will pursue the Coalition Agreement and policies announced in the Budget on 22 June in relation to public sector pay restraint.

4.36 Pay decisions should be led by healthcare employers rather than imposed by the Government. In future, all individual employers will have the right, as foundation trusts have now, to determine pay for their own staff. However, it is likely that many providers will want to continue to use national contracts as a basis for their local terms and conditions. In the short term, the Budget announced that pay will be frozen for two years for those earning more than £21,000 and the Government will ask the Pay Review Bodies to make recommendations on pay for those earning below this threshold, with a minimum increase of £250 for each year of the freeze. In the longer term, we will work with NHS employers and trade unions to explore appropriate arrangements for setting pay. However, while ministers will retain responsibility for determining overall resources and affordability, we would expect employers to take the lead in providing advice on staffing and cost pressures. Employers would also be responsible for leading negotiations on new employment contracts. In line with our aim of a decentralised system, the main incentives for financial management and efficiency will in future come from tariff-setting and a transparent regulatory framework – not from central government controls on providers' pay and internal processes.

NHS pensions

4.37   The Government has announced that Lord John Hutton will chair an independent review of public pensions, including those in the NHS. This wide ranging review will look not only at the affordability and sustainability of public service pensions but will also consider issues such as access, the impact on labour market mobility between the public and private sectors, and the extent to which pensions may act as a barrier to greater plurality of provision of public services. We will consider the findings of that review in due course but remain committed to ensuring that pension solutions are found that are fair to the workforce in the health service and fair to the taxpayer.

5.   Cutting bureaucracy and improving efficiency

5.1   The Government has guaranteed that health spending will increase in real terms in every year of this Parliament. With that protection comes the same obligation for the NHS to cut waste and transform productivity as applies to other parts of the public sector.

5.2   This discipline is also required to meet the costs of demographic change and new technologies. Since its inception, the NHS budget has risen by an average of over 4% in real terms each year; so even with our spending commitment, the NHS will face a sustained and substantial financial constraint. We will not cut the NHS as happened in the 1970s in a previous financial crisis. Meeting this challenge will require difficult local decisions, and that would be true under any government. The scale of the NHS productivity challenge may prompt calls during this Parliament for even bigger increases in NHS resources; but the reality is that there is no more money.

Cutting bureaucracy and administrative costs

5.3   So our first task is to increase the proportion of resource available for front-line services, by cutting the costs of health bureaucracy. Over the past decade, layers of national and regional organisations have accumulated, resulting in excessive bureaucracy, inefficiency and duplication. The Government will therefore impose the largest reduction in administrative costs in NHS history. Over the next four years we will reduce the NHS's management costs by more than 45%.

5.4   Reduction on this scale cannot be met by cutting all organisations equally; instead, it can only be realised by radically simplifying the architecture of the health and care system. The Government's plans for decentralisation, set out in the previous chapter, will bring major savings. PCTs – with administrative costs of over a billion pounds a year – and practice-based commissioners, will together be replaced by GP consortia. The Department will radically reduce its own NHS functions. Strategic health authorities will be abolished.

5.5   The Department will shortly publish a review of its arm's-length bodies. Subject to Parliamentary approval, we will abolish organisations that do not need to exist. We will streamline those functions that need to remain, to cut cost and remove duplication and burdens on the NHS. In future, the Department will impose tight governance over the costs and scope of all its arm's-length bodies. For example, to prevent duplication and aid transparency, the Secretary of State will consider, for any particular arm's-length body, setting out an explicit list of functions that it is not to undertake, to complement the positive list of what it is expected to do. In future, quangos' independence will be about how they perform clear and agreed functions, not the freedom to assume new roles.

5.6 The Government does not embark upon these changes lightly. Taken together, they amount to a major delayering, which will cause significant disruption and loss of jobs, and incur transitional costs between now and 2013, even as we are cutting the management cost of the NHS. But it has rapidly become clear to us that the NHS simply cannot continue to afford to support the costs of the existing bureaucracy; and the Government has a moral obligation to release as much money as possible into supporting front-line care.

5.7 At present, there are over 260,000 data returns[32] to the Department of Health. Later this year, the Department will initiate a fundamental review of data returns, with the aim of culling returns of limited value. This will ensure that the NHS information revolution described in chapter 2 is fuelled by data that are meaningful to patients and clinicians when making decisions about care, rather than by what has been collected historically. We will consult on the findings prior to implementation.

5.8 The Government will cut the bureaucracy involved in medical research. We have asked the Academy of Medical Sciences to conduct an independent review of the regulation and governance of medical research. In the light of this review we will consider the legislation affecting medical research, and the bureaucracy that flows from it, and bring forward plans for radical simplification.

5.9 As a further measure to support front-line services, the Department of Health will apply cuts to its budgets for centrally managed programmes, such as consultancy services and advertising spend. NHS services will increasingly be empowered to be the customers of a more plural system of IT and other suppliers.

5.10 We are moving to a system of control based on quality and economic regulation, commissioning and payments by results, rather than national and regional management. Within that context, we are committed to reducing the overall burdens of regulation across the health and social care sectors. We will therefore undertake a wide-ranging review of all health and social care regulation, with a view to making significant reductions.

5.11 The reforms outlined in this White Paper will themselves have one-off costs. We will ensure these are affordable within the requirements of the wider Spending Review, while ensuring funding is focused on front-line patient care.

Increasing NHS productivity and quality

5.12 The reforms in this White Paper will provide the NHS with greater incentives to increase efficiency and quality:

- Patients will be more involved in making decisions about their own health and care, improving outcomes and reducing costs.

- Patient choice will reward the most efficient, high quality services, reducing expenditure on less efficient care.

- The NHS information revolution will also lead to more efficient ways of providing care, such as on-line consultations. Greater transparency will make it easier to compare the performance of commissioners and providers.

- Prices will be calculated on the basis of the most efficient, high quality services rather than average cost.

- Payment will depend on quality of care and outcomes, not just volume. Penalties for poor quality will encourage providers to get care right first time.

- The NHS will be freed from inefficient micromanagement of meeting targets like the 98% requirement for A&E waits, and associated performance management bureaucracy.

- Commissioners and providers will focus on implementing best practice to achieve improvements in outcomes, supported by a comprehensive library of NICE standards, the work of the NHS Commissioning Board, model contracts and continued research.

- GP consortia will align clinical decisions in general practice with the financial consequences of those decisions.

- Local authorities' new functions will help unlock efficiencies across the NHS, social care and public health through stronger joint working.

- Existing providers will be set free and will be in charge of their own destiny, without central or regional management or support. This will be supported by a system of economic regulation overseen by Monitor that will drive efficiency. It will include a rules-based special administration regime. Hidden bail-outs will end.

5.13 Taken together, these ten changes will bring about a revolution in NHS efficiency. In the long term, they will help put the NHS on a more sustainable and resilient financial footing. The Department recognises that full implementation will take time; in particular the migration away from current risk pooling arrangements across SHAs.

Enhanced financial controls

5.14 As well as providing incentives for greater efficiency, the new arrangements will provide for enhanced financial control:

How the NHS will manage its resources

- NHS services will continue to be funded by the taxpayer. The Department of Health will receive funding voted by Parliament, and will remain accountable to Parliament and HM Treasury for NHS spend.

- The NHS Commissioning Board will be accountable to the Department for living within an annual NHS revenue limit, and subject to clear financial rules. This arrangement will introduce greater financial transparency between the Government and the NHS. The NHS Commissioning Board will allocate resources to GP consortia on the basis of need.

- GP consortia will have a high level of freedom; but in return they will be accountable to the NHS Commissioning Board for managing public funds. They will be subject to transparent controls and incentives for financial performance, and will enjoy a clear relationship with their constituent practices. Consortia will be required to take part in risk-pooling arrangements overseen by the NHS Commissioning Board; the Government will not bail out commissioners who fail. Regulations will specify a failure regime for commissioners.

- Commissioners will be free to buy services from any willing provider; and providers will compete to provide services. Providers who wish to provide NHS-funded services must be licensed by Monitor, who will assess financial viability.

- Providers of essential services may be required to take part in risk-pooling arrangements to ensure that, if a provider becomes financially unsustainable, Monitor will be able to step in and keep essential services running, without recourse to the Department of Health. The Government will not provide additional funding for failing providers. Monitor will be able to allow transparent subsidies where these are objectively justified, and agreed by commissioners.

Making savings during the transition

5.15 We will implement the reforms in this White Paper as rapidly as is possible. But the NHS cannot wait for them all to be in place to begin to deliver improvements in quality and productivity. Patients are rightly demanding the former, and the national economic position requires the latter.

5.16　The NHS has understood for some time the need to make extremely challenging improvements in productivity and efficiency. Work has begun to release £15-20 billon of efficiency savings for reinvestment across the system over the next four years whilst driving up quality. Achieving this ambition will be extremely challenging, but it is essential; and it will be given a boost by our reforms as they come on stream.

5.17　The existing Quality, Innovation, Productivity and Prevention (QIPP) initiative will continue with even greater urgency, but with a stronger focus on general practice leadership. The QIPP initiative is identifying how efficiencies can be driven and services redesigned to achieve the twin aims of improved quality and efficiency. Work has started on implementing what is required, for example by improving care for stroke patients, the "productive ward programme", increased self-care and the use of new technologies for people with long-term conditions.[33] Further efficiencies can, and need to, be made from improving energy efficiency and developing more sustainable forms of delivery across the NHS, for example through working with the Carbon Trust and similar bodies on carbon reduction programmes that reduce energy consumption and expenditure.

5.18　SHAs and PCTs have a current role in supporting QIPP. In discharging this, and to pave the way for the new arrangements, they should seek to devolve leadership of QIPP to emerging GP consortia and local authorities as rapidly as possible, wherever they are willing and able to take this on. The Department will require SHAs and PCTs to have an increased focus on maintaining financial control during the transition period, and they will also be supported in this task by Monitor. The Department will not hesitate to increase financial control arrangements during the transition, wherever that is necessary to maintain financial balance; in such instances, central control will be a necessary precursor to subsequent devolution to GP consortia.

6. Conclusion: making it happen

Engaging external organisations

6.1 This White Paper sets out the Government's strategy for liberating the NHS in the current Parliamentary term and beyond. It provides clarity of purpose: a more responsive, patient-centred NHS, which achieves outcomes that are among the best in the world. It provides certainty, through a clear policy framework to support that ambition, with increased autonomy and clear accountability at every level in the NHS.

6.2 Much work now needs to be undertaken over the next two to three years, both to manage the transition, as well as to flesh out the policy details. The Department will take this forward in partnership with external organisations, seeking their help and expertise in developing proposals that work in practice, for example on shared decision-making and choice.

6.3 The implementation of all these reforms, and the detailed approach we take, will be subject to broad consultation – with local government, patients and the public, as well as external organisations. The Government will formally consult wherever it is appropriate to do so, for example on strengthening the NHS Constitution, and on draft regulations.

6.4 The Government will shortly publish more detailed documents seeking views on commissioning for patients (the implementation of the NHS Commissioning Board and GP consortia); local democratic legitimacy in health; freeing providers and economic regulation; and the NHS outcomes framework. The report of the arm's-length bodies review will also be published shortly. Later this year, the Government will also publish for consultation a NHS information strategy, and a document on the move to a provider-led education and training system.

6.5 To support the ownership of the strategy within the NHS and to inform the implementation of this White Paper, the Department of Health will carry out a series of consultation activities with: patients, their representative groups and the public; NHS staff, their representative and professional bodies; local government; and the voluntary, social enterprise and independent sectors. This will run in parallel to the formal consultation on the proposals above.

6.6 We will need to ensure, through our consultation exercises and broader policy work, that the system is financially sustainable through the transition, as well as in the longer term. The proper management of financial risk will be of particular importance.

Proposals for legislation

6.7   Many of the changes in this White Paper require primary legislation. The Queen's Speech included a major Health Bill in the legislative programme for this first Parliamentary session. The Government will introduce this in the autumn. The principal legislative reforms will include:

- Enabling the creation of a **Public Health Service**, with a lead role on public health evidence and analysis;

- Transferring **local health improvement functions** to local authorities, with ring-fenced funding and accountability to the Secretary of State for Health;

- Placing the **Health and Social Care Information Centre**, currently a Special Health Authority, on a firmer statutory footing, with powers over other organisations in relation to information collection;

- Enshrining **improvement in healthcare outcomes** as the central purpose of the NHS;

- Making the **National Institute for Health and Clinical Excellence** a non-departmental public body, to define its role and functions, reform its processes, secure its independence, and extend its remit to social care;

- Establishing the independent **NHS Commissioning Board**, accountable to the Secretary of State, paving the way for the abolition of SHAs. The NHS Commissioning Board will initially be established as a Special Health Authority; the Bill will convert it into an independent non-departmental public body;

- Placing **clear limits on the role of the Secretary of State** in relation to the NHS Commissioning Board, and local NHS organisations, thereby strengthening the NHS Constitution;

- Giving **local authorities new functions** to increase the local democratic legitimacy in relation to the local strategies for NHS commissioning, and support integration and partnership working across social care, the NHS and public health;

- Establishing a statutory framework for a **comprehensive system of GP consortia**, paving the way for the abolition of PCTs;

- Establishing **HealthWatch** as a statutory part of the Care Quality Commission to champion services users and carers across health and social care, and turning Local Involvement Networks into local

HealthWatch;

- Reforming the **foundation trust** model, removing restrictions and enabling new governance arrangements, increasing transparency in their functions, repealing foundation trust deauthorisation and enabling the abolition of the NHS trust model;

- Strengthening the role of the **Care Quality Commission** as an effective quality inspectorate; and

- Developing **Monitor** into the economic regulator for health and social care, including provisions for special administration.

Associated with these changes, reducing the number of **arm's-length bodies** in the health sector, and amending their roles and functions.

6.8   We are clear about the coherent strategy, and we will engage people in understanding this and its implications. We are consulting on how best to implement these changes. In particular, the Department would welcome comments on the implementation of the proposals requiring primary legislation, and will publish a response to the views raised on the White Paper and the associated papers, prior to the introduction of the Bill. Comments should be sent by 5th October 2010, to:

NHSWhitePaper@dh.gsi.gov.uk

or:

White Paper team
Room 601
Department of Health
79 Whitehall
London SW1A 2NS

Managing the transition

6.9   *Liberating the NHS* involves change at every level of the NHS. The policy and legislative framework is just the start. Effective implementation will require a major and sustained implementation effort right across the NHS over a number of years. Change will happen bottom-up, for example by GP consortia having greater say and responsibility as rapidly as possible, and NHS trusts applying for foundation trust status at the earliest opportunity - rather than waiting until 2013. The pace of change will therefore vary across the country according to organisations' readiness to assume their new functions.

6.10 Alongside the White Paper, the Department is issuing a framework for managing the initial steps of the transition. This will include the principles and the values that the Department will hold itself to, to ensure that the transition is managed fairly and transparently, and in a way that respects staff and the contribution they make. Some organisations will disappear as we simplify NHS administration, and free resources to support front-line services. But the need for good managers performing essential functions, such as managing finance and contracts, will remain. There will be opportunities for managers to start new roles, and help build a more innovative and responsive NHS, for example supporting GP consortia, and within the NHS Commissioning Board.

Timetable for action

6.11 The high level timetable below outlines the Government's proposed timetable (subject to Parliamentary approval for legislation).

Commitment	Date
Further publications on: • framework for transition • NHS outcomes framework • commissioning for patients • local democratic legitimacy in health • freeing providers and economic regulation	July 2010
Report of the arm's length bodies review published	Summer 2010
Health Bill introduced in Parliament	Autumn 2010
Further publications on: • vision for adult social care • information strategy • patient choice • a provider-led education and training • review of data returns	By end 2010
Separation of SHAs' commissioning and provider oversight functions	
Public Health White Paper	Late 2010

Commitment	Date
Introduction of choice for: • care for long-term conditions • diagnostic testing, and post-diagnosis	From 2011
White Paper on social care reform	2011
Choice of consultant-led team	By April 2011
Shadow NHS Commissioning Board established as a special health authority	April 2011
Arrangements to support shadow health and wellbeing partnerships begin to be put in place	
Quality accounts expanded to all providers of NHS care	
Cancer Drug Fund established	
Choice of treatment and provider in some mental health services	From April 2011
Improved outcomes from NHS Outcomes Framework	
Expand validity, collection and use of PROMs	
Develop pathway tariffs for use by commissioners	
Quality accounts: nationally comparable information published	June 2011
Report on the funding of long-term care and support	By July 2011
Hospitals required to be open about mistakes	Summer 2011
GP consortia established in shadow form	2011/12
Tariffs: • Adult mental health currencies developed • National currencies introduced for critical care • Further incentives to reduce avoidable readmissions • Best-practice tariffs introduced for interventional radiology, day-case surgery for breast surgery, hernia repairs, and some orthopaedic surgery	2011/12
NHS Outcomes Framework fully implemented	By April 2012

Commitment	Date
Majority of reforms come into effect: • NHS Commissioning Board fully established • New local authority health and wellbeing boards in place • Limits on the ability of the Secretary of State to micromanage and intervene • Public record of all meetings between the Board and the Secretary of State • Public Health Service in place, with ring-fenced budget and local health improvement led by Directors of Public Health in local authorities • NICE put on a firmer statutory footing • HealthWatch established • Monitor established as economic regulator	April 2012
International Classification of Disease (ICD) 10 clinical diagnosis coding system introduced	From 2012/13
NHS Commissioning Board makes allocations for 2013/14 direct to GP consortia	Autumn 2012
Free choice of GP practice	2012
Formal establishment of all GP consortia	
SHAs are abolished	2012/13
GP consortia hold contracts with providers	April 2013
PCTs are abolished	From April 2013
All NHS trusts become, or are part of, foundation trusts	2013/14
All providers subject to Monitor regulation	
Choice of treatment and provider for patients in the vast majority of NHS-funded services	By 2013/14
Introduction of value-based approach to the way that drug companies are paid for NHS medicines	
NHS management costs reduced by over 45%	By end 2014
NICE expected to produce 150 quality standards	By July 2015

Glossary

Commissioning – the process of assessing the needs of a local population and putting in place services to meet those needs.

Commissioning for Quality and Innovation (CQUIN) framework – the CQUIN framework enables those commissioning care to pay for better quality care, helping promote a culture of continuous improvement.

Currencies – in a tariff-based payment system, payments are made for defined units of healthcare (such as an out-patient appointment with a consultant). These are known as currencies.

Foundation trusts – NHS providers who achieve foundation trust status have greater freedoms and are subject to less central control, enabling them to be more responsive to the needs of local populations.

Health Bill – proposals for a Health Bill were included in the Queen's Speech for the first Parliamentary session of the coalition Government. The Health Bill will bring forward the legislative changes required for the implementation of the proposals in this White Paper.

Law Commission – an independent body set up by Parliament to review and recommend reform of the law in England and Wales.

Local Involvement Networks (LINks) – LINks are local organisations in each local authority area set up to represent views of local people on health and social care services. These will become local HealthWatch. Further details are in paragraphs 2.23 to 2.25

National Clinical Audit – Assesses the quality of patient care across all NHS providers by measuring activities and outcomes, using that information to stimulate clinicians to improve their performance, to help patients choose providers, to guide commissioners, and to support regulation and performance management.

National Institute of Health and Clinical Excellence (NICE) – an independent organisation which provides advice and guidelines on the cost and effectiveness of drugs and treatments.

NHS Constitution – the NHS Constitution describes the principles and values of the NHS in England, and the rights and responsibilities of patients, the public and staff.

NHS Operating Framework – the Operating Framework sets out the priorities for the NHS for each financial year. The Government published a revised Operating Framework for this year on 21st June 2010.

Patient Reported Outcome Measures (PROMs) – PROMSprovide information on how patients feel about their own health, and the impact of the treatment or care they receive.

Pay Review Bodies - independent bodies which make recommendations on public sector pay in the light of evidence submitted by the Government, employers, staff and others.

Payment by Results – provides a transparent system for paying providers of healthcare services. By using the tariff and currencies to link payment to activity the system is designed to reward efficiency and support patient choice.

Personal health budget – an extension of personalised care planning, that gives people more choice and control over the services they receive by giving them more control over the money that is spent on their care.

Primary care trusts (PCTs) – the NHS body currently responsible for commissioning healthcare services and, in most cases, providing community-based services such as district nursing, for a local area.

Provider – organisations which provide services direct to patients, including hospitals, mental health services and ambulance services.

Quality accounts – a report on the quality of services published annually by providers of NHS care. Quality accounts are intended to enhance accountability to the public.

Spending Review – the Spending Review will set out the Government's priorities, and spending plans to meet these priorities, for the period 2011/12 to 2014/15.

Strategic health authorities (SHAs) – the 10 public bodies which currently oversee commissioning and provision of NHS services at a regional level.

Tariff – in relation to payment by results, the tariff it the calculated price for a unit of healthcare activity.

Value-based pricing – a mechanism for ensuring patients can get access to the medicines they need by linking the prices the NHS pays drug providers to the value of the treatment.

Venous thromboembolism (VTE) – a condition in which a blood clot (thrombus) forms in a vein. An embolism occurs if all or a part of the clot breaks off from the site where it forms and travels through the venous system.

Notes

[1] This White Paper applies only to the NHS in England. The devolved administrations in Scotland, Wales and Northern Ireland are responsible for developing their own health policies.

[2] European Union and domestic legislation prohibit discrimination on a number of grounds at work or in employment services, when providing goods, facilities or services to the public or disposing of or managing premises, in relation to education, when exercising public functions and by associations. The Equality Act 2010 which received Royal Assent on 8th April 2010 will replace existing anti-discrimination laws with one single Act and prohibit discrimination on a number of grounds such as sex, race, disability, age, religion or belief, sexual orientation, gender reassignment, pregnancy and maternity, and marriage and civil partnership.

[3] Section 6 Health Act 2009 places a duty on the Secretary of State to publish a report every three years on how the NHS Constitution has affected patients, staff, carers and members of the public, with the first report by 5 July 2012.

[4] For example, the Secretary of State has power in section 7 of the NHS Act 2006 to delegate functions to NHS bodies (other than NHS foundation trusts) and power in section 8 to direct those bodies as to the exercise of their functions. The Secretary of State also has powers to require information from NHS bodies, powers in relation to the allocation of their funding and various powers to intervene in certain NHS bodies.

[5] National Cancer Research Network, National Institute for Health Research, www.ncrn.org.uk

[6] Nolte, E., McKee, C.M, *Measuring the Health of Nations: analysis of mortality amenable to healthcare.* BMJ 2003; 327:1129; (2003).

[7] EUROCARE-4, www.eurocare.it

[8] OECD *In-hospital case-fatality rates within 30 days after admission for ischemic stroke (2007)*

[9] OECD, *Health at a Glance 2009,* (2009).

[10] OECD, *Health at a Glance 2009*, (2009).

[11] European Antimicrobial Resistance Surveillance System (EARSS) incidence of MRSA per 100,000 patient days (2008).

[12] House of Commons Health Committee. *The prevention of venous thromboembolism in hospitalised patients.* Second report of session 2004-5. (2007).

[13] *Freedom Fairness Responsibility: The Coalition: our programme for government,* www.cabinetoffice.gov.uk/media/409088/pfg_coalition.pdf

[14] Chote, R., Crawford, R., Emmerson, C., Tetlow, G., *Britain's Fiscal Squeeze: the Choices Ahead,* Institute for Fiscal Studies (2009).

[15] World Health Organization defines a high performing health system as one that should be "responsive to people's needs and preferences, treating them with dignity and respect when they come in contact with the system", *The Tallinn Charter: Health Systems for Health and Wealth Draft Charter.* WHO, (2008).

Goodrich, J., and Cornwell, J., *Seeing the person in the patient: the Point of Care,* The King's Fund (2008).

[16] "There is a need for significant progress to improve issues such as the provision of information, noise in hospitals, and the engagement of patients in decisions about their care", Richards, N., and Coulter, A., *Is the NHS becoming more patient centred? Trends from the national surveys of patients in England 2002-2007,* Picker Institute (2007).

[17] Fremont, A.M., et al 'Patient-centred processes of care and long-term outcomes of myocardial infarction.' *Journal of General Internal Medicine* 16: pp.800-8, (2001).

Bechel, D.L., Myers, W.A., Smith, D.G., 'Does patient-centred care pay off?' *Joint Commission Journal of Quality Improvement* 26(7): pp.400-9, (2000).

Kaplan, S.H., Greenfield, S., Ware, J.E., 'Assessing the effects of physician-patient interactions on the outcomes of chronic disease' *Medical Care* 27(3)Suppl: pp.S110-27, (1989).

[18] Stevenson, F.A., Cox, K., Britten, N., Dundar, Y., 'A systematic review of the research on communication between patients and health care professionals about medicines: the consequences for concordance' *Health Expectations* 7(3): pp. 235-45, (2004).

'The Human factor: How transforming healthcare to involve the public can save money and save lives', NESTA (2010).

Garcia-Alamino, J.M., Ward, A.M., Alonso-Coello, P., Perera, R., Bankhead, C., Fitzmaurice, D., Heneghan, C.J., 'Self-monitoring and self-management of oral anticoagulation', *Cochrane Database of Systematic Reviews*, Issue 4 (2010).

[19] One of the three future scenarios modelled in the report was a "fully engaged" scenario where patients and the public were more engaged in their health, contributing to significantly lower demands on the health service in the longer-term. Wanless, D., *Securing our Future Health: Taking a Long-Term View*, (2002).

[20] Heisler, M., Bouknight, R.R., Hayward, R.A., Smith, D.M., Kerr, E.A., 'The relative importance of physician communication, participatory decision-making, and patient understanding in diabetes self-management' *Journal of General Internal Medicine* 17(4): pp.243-52, (2002).

[21] Hibbard, Judith, H., Stockard, Jean, Tusler, Martin. *Hospital performance reports : impact on quality, market share, and reputation,* Health Affairs, vol 24, no 4, p 1150-1160, (2005).

Radcliffe, Bate, P., Robert G., *Bringing User Experience to Healthcare Improvement.* (2007).

[22] The 2009 British Social Attitudes Survey shows that over 95% of people think that there should be at least some choice over which hospital a patient attends and what kind of treatment they receive.

[23] Centre for Healh Economics, *Evaluation of the London Patient Choice project system wide impacts*, University of York (2004).

[24] *The Report on the National Patient Choice Survey* (2009) shows only 47% of patients being offered choice. This is confirmed by the King's Fund report *How patients choose and how providers respond*, (2010), which showed that 49% of patients recall being offered choice.

[25] www.nice.org.uk/aboutnice/qualitystandards/vteprevention/

[26] Department of Health, *Guidance on the NHS Standard Contract for Acute Services, 2010/11.*

[27] National services are defined each year in Regulations, currently there are 52. Examples include: heart and liver transplants. www.opsi.gov.uk/si/si2010/uksi_20100405_en_1

[28] Regional services (34 in all) are defined in the Specialised Services National Definition Set (SSNDS). Examples include spinal injuries, specialised cancer care, burn care and bone marrow transplantation. www.ncg.nhs.uk/index.php/key-documents/specialised-services-national-definitions-set/

[29] Sections 65A to 65Z3 of the NHS Act 2006.

[30] See, for example, the description of how concurrency works between Ofcom and OFT, set out on Ofcom's website at www.ofcom.org.uk/about/accoun/oft/

[31] Boorman, S., *The Final Report of the independent NHS Health and Well-being review*, (2009).

Department of Health, *NHS health and well-being review – the government response*, (2009).

[32] Data from an analysis of the total number of returns submitted each year to the Department of Health from NHS Trusts, PCTsPCTs and Strategic Health Authorities based on June 2010 data.

[33] *NHS Evidence QIPP Specialist Library,* www.evidence.nhs.uk/aboutus/Pages/AboutQIPP.aspx

Department of Health, *Impact Assessment for Implementing Personalised Care Planning for People with Long Term Conditions (including guidance to NHS and Social Care),* (2009).

Department of Health, *Research evidence on the effectiveness of self care support*, (2007).

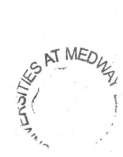